Preface

The standardized Auricular Acupuncture Point was drawn up by the World Federation of Acupuncture–Moxibustion Societies. In addition to the main body, there are three referential annexes, namely A, B and C.

Supporting institutions: Beijing University of Traditional Chinese Medicine, China Academy of Chinese Medical Sciences.

Main drafters: Zhao Baixiao, Zhou Liqun.

International members of the working group: Huang Lichun (America), Terry Oleson (America), Lao Lixing (America), Hamid Abdi (Iran), Liu Shanshan (China), Wang Xiaohong (China), Wang Lei (China), Meng Xiaonan (China).

International observers: Ma Ying (China).

1 Scope

International standards for AAP nomenclature and location.

These standards can be applied to AAP nomenclature and location.

2 Terms and Definitions

2.1 Positional Nomenclature

2.1.1 Front of the Auricle

The anterolateral side of the auricle.

2.1.2 Back of the Auricle

The posteromedial side of the auricle.

2.1.3 Anterior

The aspect of the auricle near the cheek.

2.1.4 Posterior

The aspect of the auricle near the occiput.

2.1.5 Superior

The aspect of the auricle toward the top of the skull.

2.1.6 Inferior

The aspect of the auricle toward the foot.

2.1.7 Medial

The side of the auricle proximal to the median sagittal plane.

2.1.8 Lateral

The side of the auricle distal to the median sagittal plane.

2.2 Anatomical Nomenclature

2.2.1 The Anterior Surface

2.2.1.1 Lobe

2.2.1.1.1 Lobe

The lowest part of the auricle; devoid of cartilage.

2.2.1.1.2 Anterior Groove of the Ear Lobe

The groove between the lobe and the cheek.

2.2.1.2 Helix

2.2.1.2.1 Helix

The prominent, curved, free rim of the auricle.

2.2.1.2.2 Helix Crus

A transverse ridge of the helix that continues posteriorly into the ear cavity.

2.2.1.2.3 Spine of the Helix Crus

Between anthelix and helicis uplift.

2.2.1.2.4 Notch of the Helix Crus

The cartilaginous prominence between the helix and the helix crus.

2.2.1.2.5 Helix Tubercle

The small prominence located on the posterior–superior portion of the helix.

2.2.1.2.6 Helix Cauda

The inferior part of the helix at the junction of the helix and the lobe.

2.2.1.2.7 Helix–Lobe Notch

The depression between the helix and the posterior rim of the lobe.

2.2.1.2.8 Anterior Groove of the Helix

The groove formed by the connection between the helix and the cheek.

2.2.1.3 Antihelix

2.2.1.3.1 Antihelix

The "Y" shape prominence, roughly opposite the helix, formed by the body of the antihelix, the superior antihelix crus, and the inferior antihelix crus.

2.2.1.3.2 Body of Antihelix

The principal, rough and vertical part of the antihelix.

2.2.1.3.3 Superior Antihelix Crus

The superior branch of the bifurcation of the antihelix.

2.2.1.3.4 Inferior Antihelix Crus

The inferior branch of the bifurcation of the antihelix.

2.2.1.3.5 Antihelix–Antitragus Notch

The depression between the antihelix and antitragus.

2.2.1.4 Scapha

The curved depression between the helix and the antihelix; the scaphoid fossa.

2.2.1.5 Triangular Fossa

The triangular depression bordered by the two antihelix crura and the helix.

2.2.1.6 Concha

2.2.1.6.1 Concha

The hollow area borders the orifice of the external auditory meatus. It is bordered by the helix, the antihelix, the tragus, and the antitragus; composed of the cymba conchae and the cavum conchae.

2.2.1.6.2 Cymba Conchae

The part of the concha superior to the helix crus.

2.2.1.6.3 Cavum Conchae

The part of the concha inferior to the helix crus.

2.2.1.7 Tragus

2.2.1.7.1 Tragus

The curved cartilaginous flap projecting lateral to the external auditory meatus.

2.2.1.7.2 Supratragic Notch

The depression between the tragus and the lower border of the helix crus.

2.2.1.7.3 Apex of the Upper Tragus

The superior prominence on the free rim of the tragus.

2.2.1.7.4 Apex of the Lower Tragus

The inferior prominence on the free rim of the tragus.

2.2.1.7.5 Anterior Groove of the Tragus

The shallow groove between the tragus and the cheek.

2.2.1.8 Antitragus

2.2.1.8.1 Antitragus

The flap opposite the tragus and superior to the ear lobe.

2.2.1.8.2 Apex of the Antitragus

The point at the free end of the antitragus.

2.2.1.8.3 Intertragic Notch

The depression between the tragus and antitragus.

2.2.1.9 Orifice of the External Auditory Meatus

The foramen anterior to the cavum conchae.

2.2.2 Posterior Surface of the Auricle

2.2.2.1 Back of the Helix

The flat area on the posteromedial surface of the auricle formed by the helix.

2.2.2.2 Back of the Helix Cauda

The flat area on the posteromedial surface of the auricle formed by the helix cauda.

2.2.2.3 Back of the Ear Lobe

The flat area on the posteromedial surface of the ear lobe.

2.2.2.4 Prominence of the Scapha

The prominence formed by the scapha on the posteromedial surface of the auricle.

2.2.2.5 Prominence of the Triangular Fossa

The prominence formed by the triangular fossa on the posteromedial surface of the auricle.

2.2.2.6 Prominence of the Cymba Conchae

The prominence formed by the cymba conchae on the posteromedial surface of the auricle.

2.2.2.7 Prominence of the Cavum Conchae

The prominence formed by the cavum conchae on the posteromedial surface of the auricle.

2.2.2.8 Groove of the Superior Antihelix Crus

The depression formed by the superior antihelix crus on the posteromedial surface of the auricle.

2.2.2.9 Groove of the Inferior Antihelix Crus

The depression formed by the inferior antihelix crus on the posteromedial surface of the auricle.

2.2.2.10 Groove of the Antihelix

The depression formed by the antihelix on the posteromedial surface of the auricle.

2.2.2.11 Groove of the Helix Crus

The depression formed by the helix crus on the posteromedial surface of the auricle.

2.2.2.12 Groove of the Antitragus

The depression formed by the antitragus on the posteromedial surface of the auricle.

2.2.3 Auricular Root

2.2.3.1 Superior Auricular Root

The highest part of the auricular attachment to the scalp.

2.2.3.2 Inferior Auricular Root

The lowest part of the auricular attachment where the ear lobe attaches to the cheek.

3 An Introduction to AAP Nomenclature and Location

The following introduction is applicable to AAP nomenclature and location.

a. Annex B gives the principles of AAP nomenclature and location.

b. Annex C and Figure A1 of Annex A show the basic marking lines, points, and areas of the auricle.

c. Old names, other names, and literature.

d. Written forms for AAP nomenclature and location: Chinese name, Chinese pinyin, code and point location are supplied.

e.AAP names and locations are shown in Figures A2 and A3 of Annex A.

4 Names and Locations of AAPs

4.1 Points on the Helix

4.1.1 Ear Center ěrzhōng (HX$_1$)

HX$_1$ is located on the helix crus.

4.1.2 Rectum zhícháng (HX$_2$)

HX$_2$ is located on the helix anterior to the helix crus.

4.1.3 Urethra niàodào (HX$_3$)

HX$_3$ is located on the helix superior to zhichang (HX$_2$).

4.1.4 External Genitals wàishēngzhíqì (HX$_4$)

HX$_4$ is located on the helix anterior to the helix crus.

4.1.5 Anus gāngmén (HX$_5$)

HX$_5$ is located on the helix anterior to the triangular fossa.

4.1.6 Anterior Ear Apex ěrjiānqiánqū (HX$_6$)

HX$_6$ is located anterior to the ear apex.

4.1.7 Ear Apex ěrjiān (HX$_{6,7i}$)

HX$_{6,7i}$ is the apex formed when the auricle is folded anteriorly at the juncture of HX$_6$ and HX$_7$.

4.1.8 Posterior Ear Apex ěrjiānhòuqū (HX$_7$)

HX$_7$ is posterior to the ear apex.

4.1.9 Node jiéjié (HX$_8$)

HX$_8$ is located on the helix at the helix tuberclev.

4.1.10 Helix 1 lúnyī (HX$_9$)

HX$_9$ is located on the inferior border of the helix.

4.1.11 Helix 2 lúnèr (HX$_{10}$)

HX$_{10}$ is located on the helix inferior to HX$_1$.

4.1.12 Helix 3 lúnsān (HX$_{11}$)

HX$_{11}$ is located on the helix inferior to HX$_2$.

4.1.13 Helix 4 lúnsì (HX$_{12}$)

HX$_{12}$ is on the helix inferior to HX$_3$.

4.2 Points in the Scapha

4.2.1 Finger zhǐ (SF$_1$)

SF$_1$ is in the superior scapha.

4.2.2 Wrist wàn (SF$_2$)

SF$_2$ is in the area inferior to SF$_1$.

4.2.3 Windstream fēngxī (SF$_{1,2i}$)

SF$_{1,2i}$ is located in the area anterior to the helix tubercle at the juncture of SF$_1$ and SF$_2$.

4.2.4 Elbow zhǒu (SF$_3$)

SF$_3$ is located in the area inferior to SF$_2$.

4.2.5 Shoulder jiān (SF$_{4,5}$)

SF$_{4,5}$ is located in the area inferior to SF$_3$.

4.2.6 Clavicle suǒgǔ (SF$_6$)

SF$_6$ is located in the area inferior to SF$_{4,5}$.

4.3 Points on the Antihelix

4.3.1 Heel gēn (AH$_1$)

AH$_1$ is located on the anterosuperior part of the superior antihelix crus.

4.3.2 Toe zhǐ (AH$_2$)

AH$_2$ is in the posterosuperior area of the superior antihelix crus inferior to the apex.

4.3.3 Ankle huái (AH$_3$)

AH$_3$ is located on the area inferior to AH$_1$ and AH$_2$.

4.3.4 Knee xī (AH$_4$)

AH$_4$ is located on the middle 1/3rd of the superior antihelix crus.

4.3.5 Hip kuān (AH$_5$)

AH$_5$ is located on the lower 1/3rd of the superior antihelix crus.

4.3.6 Sciatic Nerve zuògǔshénjīng (AH$_6$)

AH$_6$ is located on the anterior 2/3rds of the inferior antihelix crus.

4.3.7 Sympathetic Nerve jiāogǎn (AH$_{6a}$)

AH$_{6a}$ is anterior to AH$_6$ at the juncture of the end of the inferior antihelix crus and the medial edge of the helix.

4.3.8 Gluteus tún (AH$_7$)

AH$_7$ is located on the posterior 1/3rd of the inferior antihelix crus.

4.3.9 Abdomen fù (AH$_8$)

AH$_8$ is located on the upper 2/5ths of the body of the antihelix.

4.3.10 Lumbosacral Vertebrae yāodǐzhuī (AH$_9$)

AH$_9$ is located on the body of the antihelix posterior to AH$_8$.

4.3.11 Chest xiōng (AH$_{10}$)

AH$_{10}$ is on the middle 2/5ths of the body of the antihelix.

4.3.12 Thoracic Vertebrae xiōngzhuī (AH$_{11}$)

AH$_{11}$ is located on the body of the antihelix posterior to AH$_{10}$.

4.3.13 Neck jǐng (AH$_{12}$)

AH$_{12}$ is located on the lower 1/5th of the body of the antihelix.

4.3.14 Cervical Vertebrae jǐngzhuī (AH$_{13}$)

AH$_{13}$ is located on the body of the antihelix posterior to AH$_{12}$.

4.4 Points in the Triangular Fossa

4.4.1 Superior Triangular Fossa jiǎowōshàng (TF$_1$)

TF$_1$ is located in the upper part of the superior 1/3 of the triangular fossa.

4.4.2 Internal Genitals nèishēngzhíqì (TF$_2$)

TF$_2$ is located in the lower part of the superior 1/3 of the triangular fossa.

4.4.3 Middle Triangular Fossa jiǎowōzhōng (TF$_3$)

TF$_3$ is located in the middle 1/3 of the triangular fossa.

4.4.4 Shenmen shénmén (TF$_4$)

TF$_4$ is located in the upper part of the posterior 1/3 of the triangular fossa.

4.4.5 Pelvis pénqiāng (TF₅)

TF$_5$ is located in the lower part of the posterior 1/3 of the triangular fossa.

4.5 Points on the Tragus

4.5.1 Upper Tragus shàngpíng (TG₁)

TG$_1$ is located on the upper 1/2 of the external surface of the tragus.

4.5.2 Lower Tragus xiàpíng (TG₂)

TG$_2$ is located at the lower 1/2 of the external surface of the tragus.

4.5.3 External Ear wàiěr (TG₁ᵤ)

TG$_{1u}$ is inferior to the helix crus and anterior to the supratragic notch on the upper edge of TG$_1$.

4.5.4 Apex of Tragus píngjiān (TG₁ₚ)

TG$_{1p}$ is located on the projection of the upper tragus at the posterior edge of TG$_1$.

4.5.5 External Nose wàibí (TG₁,₂ᵢ)

TG$_{1,2i}$ is located at the midpoint of the external surface of the tragus at the juncture of the TG$_1$ and TG$_2$.

4.5.6 Adrenal Gland shènshàngxiàn (TG₂ₚ)

TG$_{2p}$ is located on the end of the inferior edge of the tragus at the posterior edge of TG$_2$.

4.5.7 Pharynx and Larynx yānhóu (TG₃)

TG$_3$ is located at the upper 1/2 of the internal side of the tragus.

4.5.8 Internal Nose nèibí (TG₄)

TG$_4$ is located on the lower 1/2 of the internal side of the tragus.

4.5.9 Anterior Intertragic Notch píngjiānqián (TG₂ₗ)

TG$_{2l}$ is located at the lowest part of the front surface of the intertragic notch on the inferior edge of TG$_2$.

4.6 Points on the Antitragus

4.6.1 Forehead é (AT₁)

AT$_1$ is located in the anterior area of the lateral side of the antitragus.

4.6.2 Posterior Intertragicus píngjiānhòu (AT₁ₗ)

AT$_{1l}$ is located at the anteroinferior part of the antitragus, posterior to intertragicus and the lower edge of AT$_1$.

4.6.3 Temple niè (AT₂)

AT$_2$ is located at the middle part of the lateral side of the antitragus.

4.6.4 Occiput zhěn (AT₃)

AT$_3$ is located at the posterior part of the lateral side of the antitragus.

4.6.5 Subcortex pízhìxià (AT₄)

AT$_4$ is located on the medial side of the antitragus.

4.6.6 Apex of Antitragus duìpíngjiān (AT₁,₂,₄ᵢ)

AT$_{1,2,4i}$ is located at the free end of the apex of the antitragus at the juncture of AT$_1$, AT$_2$ and AT$_4$.

4.6.7 Central Rim yuánzhōng (AT₂,₃,₄ᵢ)

AT$_{2,3,4i}$ is located on the free rim at the midpoint of the apex of the antitragus and antihelix–antitragus notch at the juncture of AT$_2$, AT$_3$, and AT$_4$.

4.6.8 Brain Stem nǎogàn (AT₃,₄ᵢ)

AT$_{3,4i}$ is located at the antihelix–antitragus notch at the juncture of AT$_3$ and AT$_4$.

4.7 Points in the Concha

4.7.1 Mouth kǒu (CO₁)

CO$_1$ is located in the concha inferior to the anterior 1/3rd of the helix crus.

4.7.2 Esophagus shídào (CO_2)

CO_2 is located in the concha inferior to the intermediate 1/3rd of the helix crus.

4.7.3 Cardia bēnmén (CO_3)

CO_3 is located in the concha inferior to the posterior 1/3rd of the helix crus.

4.7.4 Stomach wèi (CO_4)

CO_4 is located at the end of the helix crus.

4.7.5 Duodenum shíèrzhǐcháng (CO_5)

CO_5 is located in the posterior 1/3rd of the region between the helix crus and Line AB.

4.7.6 Small Intestine xiǎocháng (CO_6)

CO_6 is located at the intermediate 1/3rd of the region between the helix crus and Line AB.

4.7.7 Large Intestine dàcháng (CO_7)

CO_7 is located at the anterior 1/3rd of the region between the helix crus and Line AB.

4.7.8 Appendix lánwěi ($CO_{6,7i}$)

$CO_{6,7i}$ is located at the juncture of CO_6 and CO_7.

4.7.9 Angle of Superior Concha tǐngjiǎo (CO_8)

CO_8 is located in the cymba conchae below the anterior region of the inferior antihelix crus.

4.7.10 Bladder pángguāng (CO_9)

CO_9 is located in the cymba conchae below the intermediate region of the inferior antihelix crus.

4.7.11 Kidney shèn (CO_{10})

CO_{10} is located in the cymba conchae below the posterior region of the inferior antihelix crus.

4.7.12 Ureter shūniàoguǎn ($CO_{9,10i}$)

$CO_{9,10i}$ is located at the juncture of CO_9 and CO_{10}.

4.7.13 Pancreas and Gallbladder yídǎn (CO_{11})

CO_{11} is located in the posterosuperior part of the cymba conchae.

4.7.14 Liver gān (CO_{12})

CO_{12} is located in the posteroinferior part of the cymba conchae.

4.7.15 Center of Superior Concha tǐngzhōng ($CO_{6,10i}$)

$CO_{6,10i}$ is located at the juncture of CO_6 and CO_{10}.

4.7.16 Spleen pí (CO_{13})

CO_{13} is located in the region inferior to line BD, posterosuperior to the cavum conchae.

4.7.17 Heart xīn (CO_{15})

CO_{15} is located in the center of the depression of the cavum conchae.

4.7.18 Trachea qìguǎn (CO_{16})

CO_{16} is located between the CO_{15} and the orifice of the external auditory meatus.

4.7.19 Lung fèi (CO_{14})

CO_{14} is located in the cavum conchae in the region surrounding CO_{15} and CO_{16}.

4.7.20 Triple Energizer sānjiāo (CO_{17})

CO_{17} is located between CO_{14} and CO_{18} in the region posteroinferior to the orifice of the external auditory meatus.

4.7.21 Endocrine nèifēnmì (CO_{18})

CO_{18} is inside of the intertragus notch in the anteroinferior region of the cavum conchae.

4.8　Points on the Ear Lobe

4.8.1　Tooth yá (LO$_1$)

LO$_1$ is located in the anterosuperior area of the anterolateral surface of the lobe.

4.8.2　Tongue shé (LO$_2$)

LO$_2$ is located in the intermediate superior area of the anterolateral surface of the lobe.

4.8.3　Jaw hé (LO$_3$)

LO$_3$ is located in the posterosuperior area of the anterolateral surface of the lobe.

4.8.4　Anterior Ear Lobe chuíqián (LO$_4$)

LO$_4$ is in the anterior intermediate area of the anterolateral surface of the lobe.

4.8.5　Eye yǎn (LO$_5$)

LO$_5$ is in the center of the anterolateral surface of the lobe.

4.8.6　Internal Ear nèiěr (LO$_6$)

LO$_6$ is in the intermediate posterior area of the anterolateral surface of the lobe.

4.8.7　Cheek miànjiá (LO$_{5,6i}$)

LO$_{5,6i}$ is located in the intermediate posterior part of the anterolateral surface of the lobe at the juncture of LO$_5$ and LO$_6$.

4.8.8　Tonsil biǎntáotǐ (LO$_{7,8,9}$)

LO$_{7,8,9}$ are the three divisions of the inferior anterolateral surface of the lobe.

4.9　Points on the Posterior Surface of the Ear

4.9.1　Heart, Posteromedial Surface of the Ear ěrbèixīn (P$_1$)

P$_1$ is located on the superior area of the posteromedial surface of the ear.

4.9.2　Lung, Posteromedial Surface ěrbèifèi (P$_2$)

P$_2$ is on the intermediate medial area of the posteromedial surface of the ear.

4.9.3　Spleen, Posteromedial Surface ěrbèipí (P$_3$)

P$_3$ is located at the center of the posteromedial surface of the ear.

4.9.4　Liver, Posteromedial Surface ěrbèigān (P$_4$)

P$_4$ is on the intermediate lateral area of the posteromedial surface of the ear.

4.9.5　Kidney, Posteromedial Surface ěrbèishèn (P$_5$)

P$_5$ is located in the inferior area of the posteromedial surface of the ear lobe.

4.9.6　Groove, Posteromedial Surface ěrbèigōu (P$_S$)

Ps is the groove on the posteromedial surface of the ear formed by the superior and inferior antihelix crura.

4.10　Points at the Root of the Ear

4.10.1　Upper Ear Root shàngěrgēn (R$_1$)

R$_1$ is the highest point at which the ear attaches to the head.

4.10.2　Root of Ear Vagus ěrmígēn (R$_2$)

R$_2$ is located on the ear root at the posteromedial groove formed by the helix crus.

4.10.3　Lower Ear Root xiàěrgēn (R$_3$)

R$_3$ is the lowest point on the ear root.

Annex A
(Informative)
Figures

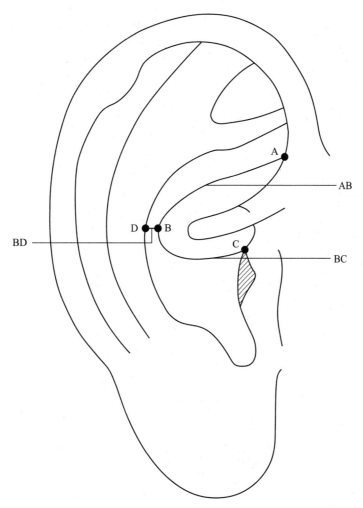

Figure A1   Supplement to the Basic Imaginary Points and Lines

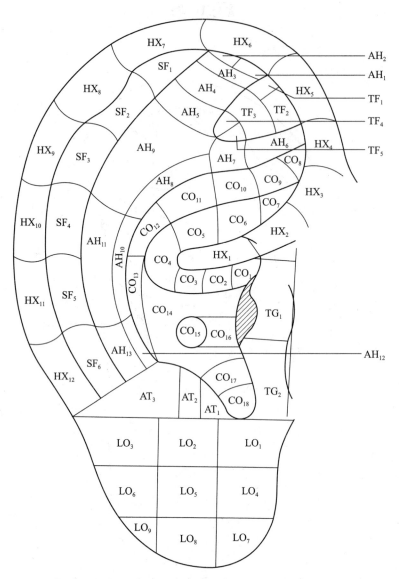

Figure A2   Standard Codes for the Divisions of the Auricle (Anterolateral)

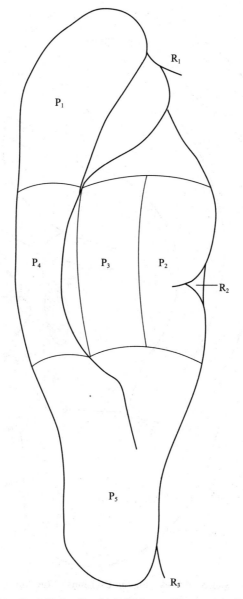

Figure A3   Standard Codes for the Divisions of the Auricle (Posteromedial)

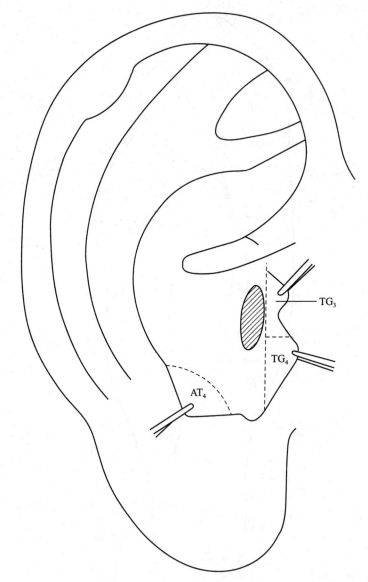

Figure A4   Standard Codes for the Divisions of the Auricle (Medial)

Annex B

(Informative)

Principles of AAP Nomenclature and Location

B.1 Principles for Including an AAP in This Standardization

B.1.1 The AAP has an extensive practical basis.

B.1.2 The AAP is commonly used.

B.1.3 The AAP has been proven diagnostic and treatment effects.

B.2 Further Principles of Inclusion

Further principles of inclusion: Named points are selected on the following bases.

B.2.1 Internationally known points or those in common use, e.g. sympathesis.

B.2.2 Points with well-proven therapeutic effects that are recorded in traditional medicine literature, e.g., windstream.

B.2.3 Points named for organs and other parts of the body, e.g. heart, shoulder.

B.2.4 Points named by anatomical features of the auricle, e.g. upper ear root, middle triangular fossa, ear apex, ear center, etc.

B.2.5 The following approach of naming points are not acceptable in this standardization:

a.Naming for a particular disease.

b.Naming according to functions of diagnosis or treatment.

c.Designations based on drug names.

d.Alternative point names not chosen for this standarization.

e.Names referring to gender.

f.Names of points that otherwise do not meet the standards of inclusion.

B.3 Principles of AAP Location

B.3.1 In this standardization, location is principally based on the anatomical divisions of the auricle.

B.3.2 Definite terms and denoting position on the auricle are used.

B.3.3 Anatomical names of features on the auricle that have connection with AAP divisions are used.

B.3.4 Imaginary points based on the anatomical topography of the auricle are also used.

B.3.5 Imaginary lines on the auricle are used to clarify the boundaries of anatomic-al structures and thus identify designated AAPs.

B.3.6 The entire surface of the auricle is mapped with named AAPs and regions.

Annex C

(Informative)

Introduction to the Basic Imaginary Points, Lines and Divisions of the Auricle

C.1   Basic Marking Line Designations on the Auricle

The following basic imaginary lines are applicable:

C.1.1   Medial Rim of the Helix

The boundary between the helix and other parts of the auricle; a fold line formed by the helix, scapha, crura of the antihelix, triangular fossa, and the concha.

C.1.2   Fold Line of the Concha

The boundary between the flat part and the prominent part of the concha.

C.1.3   Line of the Antihelix Spine

A connecting line, formed by the highest prominence stretching from the bifurcation to the body of the antihelix.

C.1.4   Line of the Groove of the Scapha

A line at the deepest depression of the scapha.

C.1.5   Boundary of the Antihelix and the Scapha

The midline between the antihelix (including the superior antihelix crus) spine and the groove of the scapha.

C.1.6   The Posterior Edge of the Triangular Fossa

The lower border of the triangular fossa.

C.1.7   Boundary of the Antihelix and the Triangular Fossa

The midline between the spine of the antihelix crura and the posterior edge of triangular fossa.

C.1.8   The Concha Edge of the Antihelix

The midline between the spine of antihelix (including the inferior antihelix crus), and the anatomical border between the antihelix and the concha.

C.1.9   The Inferior Edge of the Antihelix

The boundary between the superior antihelix crus and the body of the antihelix formed by a line extending vertically from the bifurcation of the antihelix to the boudary of the antihelix and the scapha.

C.1.10   The Posterior Edge of the Antihelix

The boundary of the inferior antihelix crus and the body of the antihelix formed by a line extending vertically from the bifurcation of the antihelix to the concha edge of the antihelix.

C.1.11   The Superior Line of the Ear Lobe

The boundary between the lobe and other parts of the auricle.

C.1.12   The Concha Edge of the Antitragus

The boundary between the medial rim of the antihelix and the concha.

C.1.13   The Anterior Edge of the Tragus

The boundary between the anterior of the tragus and the cheek.

C.1.14   The Anterior Edge of the Helix

The boundary between the helix and the cheek.

C.1.15   The Anterior Edge of the Ear Lobe

The boundary between the lobe and the cheek.

C.2   Imaginary Points and Lines on the Auricle

The following basic imaginary points and lines apply to the auricle.

C.2.1   Imaginary Point A is located at the medial edge of the helix at the junction between the middle and upper 1/3rd of the line from the notch of helix crus and the inferior edge of the inferior antihelix crus.

C.2.2   Imaginary Point D is located where a level line drawn from the end of the helix crus crosses the concha edge of the antihelix.

C.2.3   Imaginary Point B is located at the junction of the middle and posterior 1/3rd of the line extending from the end of the helix crus to Point D.

C.2.4   Imaginary Point C is located at the junction of the upper 1/4th and lower 3/4ths of the posterior edge of the orifice of the external auditory meatus.

C.2.5   Line AB is a curved line that extends from Point A to Point B and mirrors the concha edge of the antihelix.

C.2.6   Line BC is a curved line extending from Point B to Point C that mirrors the inferior edge of the helix crus.

C.3   Introduction to the Divisions of the Auricle

C.3.1   Helix

The helix is equally divided into twelve areas. The helix crus is HX_1 (Area 1 of the Helix). The part of the helix from the helix notch to the upper edge of the inferior antihelix crus is divided into three parts, HX_2, HX_3 and HX_4, counting from below to above. The area between the two antihelix crura is designated HX_5. HX_6 extends between the anterior and posterior edges of the superior antihelix crus. HX_7 extends from the apex of the ear to the upper edge of the helix tubercle. The area from the upper edge to the lower edge of the helix tubercle is HX_8. The region from the lower edge of the helix tubercle to the notch of the helix lobe is equally divided into four areas, HX_9, HX_{10}, HX_{11} and HX_{12}, from above to below respectively.

C.3.2   Scapha

The scapha is divided into six equal areas. From above to below, they are SF_1 (Area 1 of the scapha), SF_2, SF_3, SF_4, SF_5 and SF_6.

C.3.3   Antihelix

The antihelix is divided into thirteen areas. The superior antihelix crus is divided into three equal parts. The lower third is AH_5 (Area 5 of the antihelix). The middle third is AH_4, and the upper third is divided horizontally into two equal subparts, of which the lower half is AH_3. The upper half is once again divided perpendicularly into two; the posterior half is AH_2 and the anterior half is AH_1.

The inferior antihelix crus is divided into three parts. From the anterior to the posterior, the first two–thirds are AH_6; the posterior third is AH_7.

The body of the antihelix from its bifurcation to the antihelix–antitragus notch is divided into five equal parts from the superior to the inferior, and once again it is divided into the anterior (one fourth) and the posterior (three fourths) paralleling to the boundary of the antihelix and the concha. In this way, the body of the antihelix is divided into ten parts. The anterior superior two parts are AH_8; the posterior superior two parts are AH_9; the anterior intermediate two parts are AH_{10}; the posterior intermediate two parts are AH_{11}; the anterior inferior part is AH_{12}; the posterior inferior fifth is AH_{13}.

C.3.4   Triangular Fossa

The triangular fossa is divided into three equal parts from the edge of helix to the bifurcation of the antihelix. The middle third is TF_3 (Area 3 of the triangular fossa). The anterior third is further divided into three subparts: the upper third is TF_1, and the middle and lower two–thirds are TF_2. The posterior third near the bifurcation is divided into two subparts, the upper half is TF_4 and the lower half is TF_5.

C.3.5 Tragus

The tragus is divided into four areas. The external surface of the tragus is divided into two parts; the upper part is TG_1 (Area 1 of the tragus) and the lower part is TG_2.

The internal surface of the tragus is also divided into two parts, the upper of which is TG_3 and the lower of which is TG_4.

C.3.6 Antitragus

The antitragus is divided into four areas. Draw two lines, one extending vertically from the apex of the antitragus to the superior line of the ear lobe, the other vertically from the midpoint of the antitragus to the helix notch. The external surface of the antitragus is thus divided into three areas. The anterior area is AT_1 (Area 1 of the antitragus), the intermediate is AT_2, and the posterior is AT_3.

The internal surface of the antitragus is AT_4.

C.3.7 Concha

The concha is divided into eighteen areas. The part formed by the inferior edge of the helix crus and line BC (the anterior part) is divided into three equal areas, CO_1 (Area 1 of the concha), CO_2 and CO_3, from front to back.

The fan-shaped area at the end of the helix crus is CO_4.

The part formed by the superior edge of the helix crus and line AB (the anterior part) is divided into three equal areas. From the posterior to the anterior are CO_5, CO_6 and CO_7.

CO_8 is anterior to a line drawn from point C to the junction of the anterior third and the posterior two-thirds of the lower edge of the inferior antihelix crus.

The part posterior to CO_8 and superior to CO_6 and CO_7 is divided into two equal areas; the anterior is CO_9 and the posterior is CO_{10}.

The part posterior to CO_{10} and superior to line BD is also divided into two equal areas; the superior is CO_{11} and the inferior is CO_{12}.

The area marked off by a line drawn from the antihelix–antitragus notch to Point BD is CO_{13}.

Taking the midpoint of the cavum conchae as the center of a circle with a radius of half the distance from the center to line BC gives us CO_{15}.

The area between two parallel lines drawn respectively from the highest and lowest points of the orifice of the external auditory meatus to the highest and lowest points of CO_{15} is CO_{16}.

The area external to CO_{15} and CO_{16} is CO_{14}.

The area inferior to a line drawn from the lowest point of the orifice of the external auditory meatus to the midpoint of the concha edge of the antihelix is divided into two equal areas: the upper is CO_{17} and the lower is CO_{18}.

C.3.8 Lobe

The lobe is divided by two equidistant vertical lines extending from superior to inferior border. Two equidistant horizontal lines, parallel to the superior border, cross the verticals to divide the lobe into nine areas. From the anterior to the posterior the upper three areas are LO_1 (Area 1 of the lobe), LO_2 and LO_3. The middle three areas are LO_4, LO_5 and LO_6. The lower three areas are LO_7, LO_8 and LO_9.

C.3.9 Posterior Surface of the Auricle

The posterior surface of auricle is divided into five areas. Two horizontal lines passing through the back corresponding to the bifurcation of the antihelix crura and the antihelix–antitragus notch were drawn to divide the posterior surface into three parts, the upper being P_1 (Area 1 of the posterior surface of the auricle) and the lower being P_5. The middle part is divided into three equal areas. The medial area is P_2, the middle is P_3, and the lateral is P_4.

前　言

耳穴名称与定位的标准由世界针灸学会联合会制定。除了主体部分，本标准附录 A、附录 B 和附录 C 是资料性附录。

支持单位：北京中医药大学、中国中医科学院。

主要起草人：赵百孝、周立群。

国际工作组成员：Huang Lichun（美国），Terry Oleson（美国），Lao Lixing（美国），Hamid Abdi（伊朗），Liu Shanshan（中国），Wang Xiaohong（中国），Wang Lei（中国），Meng Xiaonan（中国）。

国际观察员：Ma Ying（中国）。

1 范围

本标准规定了人体耳穴的名称和耳穴的标准定位。

本标准适用于耳穴名称和定位。

2 术语和定义

2.1 耳郭方位术语

2.1.1 耳郭正面

耳郭正面，指耳郭的前外侧面。

2.1.2 耳郭背面

耳郭背面，指耳郭的后内侧面，统称耳背。

2.1.3 前方

前方，指耳郭近面颊的一侧。

2.1.4 后方

后方，指耳郭近乳突的一侧。

2.1.5 上方

上方，指耳郭近头顶的一侧。

2.1.6 下方

下方，指耳郭近肩的一侧。

2.1.7 内侧

内侧，指耳郭近正中矢状面的一侧。

2.1.8 外侧

外侧，指耳郭远正中矢状面的一侧。

2.2 耳郭表面解剖名称

2.2.1 耳郭正面

2.2.1.1 耳垂

2.2.1.1.1 耳垂

耳垂，指耳郭下部无软骨的部分。

2.2.1.1.2 耳垂前沟

耳垂前沟，指耳垂与面部之间的浅沟。

2.2.1.2 耳轮

2.2.1.2.1 耳轮

耳轮，指耳郭外侧边缘的卷曲部分。

2.2.1.2.2 耳轮脚

耳轮脚，指耳轮深入耳甲的部分。

2.2.1.2.3 耳轮脚棘

耳轮脚棘，指耳轮脚和耳轮之间的隆起。

2.2.1.2.4 耳轮脚切迹

耳轮脚切迹，指耳轮脚棘前方的凹陷处。

2.2.1.2.5 耳轮结节

耳轮结节，指耳轮外上方的膨大部分。

2.2.1.2.6 耳轮尾

耳轮尾，指耳轮向下移行于耳垂的部分。

2.2.1.2.7 轮垂切迹

轮垂切迹，指耳轮和耳垂后缘之间的凹陷处。

2.2.1.2.8 耳轮前沟

耳轮前沟，指耳轮与面部之间的浅沟。

2.2.1.3 对耳轮

2.2.1.3.1 对耳轮

对耳轮，指与耳轮相对呈"Y"字形的隆起部，由对耳轮体、对耳轮上脚和对耳轮下脚三部分组成。

2.2.1.3.2 对耳轮体

对耳轮体，指对耳轮下部呈上下走向的主体部分。

2.2.1.3.3 对耳轮上脚

对耳轮上脚，指对耳轮向上分支的部分。

2.2.1.3.4 对耳轮下脚

对耳轮下脚，指对耳轮向前分支的部分。

2.2.1.3.5 轮屏切迹

轮屏切迹，指对耳轮与对耳屏之间的凹陷处。

2.2.1.4 耳舟

耳舟，指耳轮与对耳轮之间的凹沟。

2.2.1.5 三角窝

三角窝，指对耳轮上、下脚与相应耳轮之间的三角形凹窝。

2.2.1.6 耳甲

2.2.1.6.1 耳甲

耳甲，指部分耳轮和对耳轮、对耳屏、耳屏及外耳门之间的凹窝。由耳甲艇、耳甲腔两部分组成。

2.2.1.6.2 耳甲艇

耳甲艇，指耳轮脚以上的耳甲部。

2.2.1.6.3 耳甲腔

耳甲腔，指耳轮脚以下的耳甲部。

2.2.1.7 耳屏

2.2.1.7.1 耳屏

耳屏，指耳郭前方呈瓣状的软骨隆起。

2.2.1.7.2 屏上切迹

屏上切迹，指耳屏与耳轮之间的凹陷处。

2.2.1.7.3 上屏尖

上屏尖，指耳屏游离缘上隆起部。

2.2.1.7.4 下屏尖

下屏尖，指耳屏游离缘下隆起部。

2.2.1.7.5 耳屏前沟

耳屏前沟，指耳屏与面部之间的浅沟。

2.2.1.8 对耳屏

2.2.1.8.1 对耳屏

对耳屏，指耳垂上方与耳屏相对的瓣状隆起。

2.2.1.8.2 对屏尖

对屏尖，指对耳屏游离缘隆起的顶端。

2.2.1.8.3　屏间切迹

屏间切迹，指耳屏和对耳屏之间的凹陷处。

2.2.1.9　外耳门

外耳门，指耳甲腔前方的孔窍。

2.2.2　耳郭背面

2.2.2.1　耳轮背面

耳轮背面，指耳轮背部的平坦部分。

2.2.2.2　耳轮尾背面

耳轮尾背面，指耳轮尾背部的平坦部分。

2.2.2.3　耳垂背面

耳垂背面，指耳垂背部的平坦部分。

2.2.2.4　耳舟隆起

耳舟隆起，指耳舟在耳背呈现的隆起。

2.2.2.5　三角窝隆起

三角窝隆起，指三角窝在耳背呈现的隆起。

2.2.2.6　耳甲艇隆起

耳甲艇隆起，指耳甲艇在耳背呈现的隆起。

2.2.2.7　耳甲腔隆起

耳甲腔隆起，指耳甲腔在耳背呈现的隆起。

2.2.2.8　对耳轮上脚沟

对耳轮上脚沟，指对耳轮上脚在耳背呈现的凹沟。

2.2.2.9　对耳轮下脚沟

对耳轮下脚沟，指对耳轮下脚在耳背呈现的凹沟。

2.2.2.10　对耳轮沟

对耳轮沟，指对耳轮体在耳背呈现的凹沟。

2.2.2.11　耳轮脚沟

耳轮脚沟，指耳轮脚在耳背呈现的凹沟。

2.2.2.12　对耳屏沟

对耳屏沟，指对耳屏在耳背呈现的凹沟。

2.2.3　耳根

2.2.3.1　上耳根

上耳根，指耳郭与头部相连的最上处。

2.2.3.2　下耳根

下耳根，指耳郭与头部相连的最下处。

3　耳穴名称与定位的说明

下列说明适用于耳穴名称与定位：

a. 规定耳穴名称与定位的命名原则和定位原则，见附录 B。

b. 划定耳郭基本标志线，设定耳郭标志点、线，对耳郭进行分区，见附录 C 及附录 A 的图 A1。

c. 耳穴曾用名、并用名及文献沿革。

d. 耳穴名称与定位书写格式为：耳穴中文名称→汉语拼音→穴位分区编号→定位。

e. 耳穴名称与定位见附录 A 的图 A2、图 A3。

4 耳穴名称与定位

4.1 耳轮穴位

4.1.1 耳中 ěrzhōng (HX$_1$)

耳中，在耳轮脚处，即耳轮 1 区。

4.1.2 直肠 zhícháng (HX$_2$)

直肠，在耳轮脚棘前上方的耳轮处，即耳轮 2 区。

4.1.3 尿道 niàodào (HX$_3$)

尿道，在直肠上方的耳轮处，即耳轮 3 区。

4.1.4 外生殖器 wàishēngzhíqì (HX$_4$)

外生殖器，在对耳轮下脚前方的耳轮处，即耳轮 4 区。

4.1.5 肛门 gāngmén (HX$_5$)

肛门，在三角窝前方的耳轮处，即耳轮 5 区。

4.1.6 耳尖前区 ěrjiānqiánqū (HX$_6$)

耳尖前区，在耳郭向前对折上部尖端的前部，即耳轮 6 区。

4.1.7 耳尖 ěrjiān (HX$_{6,7i}$)

耳尖，在耳郭向前对折的上部尖端处，即耳轮 6、7 区交界处。

4.1.8 耳尖后区 ěrjiānhòuqū (HX$_7$)

耳尖后区，在耳郭向前对折上部尖端的后部，即耳轮 7 区。

4.1.9 结节 jiéjié (HX$_8$)

结节，在耳轮结节处，即耳轮 8 区。

4.1.10 轮 1 lúnyī (HX$_9$)

轮 1，在耳轮结节下方的耳轮处，即耳轮 9 区。

4.1.11 轮 2 lúnèr (HX$_{10}$)

轮 2，在轮 1 区下方的耳轮处，即耳轮 10 区。

4.1.12 轮 3 lúnsān (HX$_{11}$)

轮 3，在轮 2 区下方的耳轮处，即耳轮 11 区。

4.1.13 轮 4 lúnsì (HX$_{12}$)

轮 4，在轮 3 区下方的耳轮处，即耳轮 12 区。

4.2 耳舟穴位

4.2.1 指 zhǐ (SF$_1$)

指，在耳舟上方处，即耳舟 1 区。

4.2.2 腕 wàn (SF$_2$)

腕，在指区的下方处，即耳舟 2 区。

4.2.3 风溪 fēngxī (SF$_{1,2i}$)

风溪，在耳轮结节前方，指区与腕区之间，即耳舟 1、2 区交界处。

4.2.4 肘 zhǒu (SF$_3$)

肘，在腕区的下方处，即耳舟 3 区。

4.2.5 肩 jiān (SF$_{4,5}$)

肩，在肘区的下方处，即耳舟 4、5 区。

4.2.6 锁骨 suǒgǔ (SF$_6$)

锁骨，在肩区的下方处，即耳舟 6 区。

4.3 对耳轮穴位

4.3.1 跟 gēn (AH$_1$)
跟，在对耳轮上脚前上部，即对耳轮 1 区。

4.3.2 趾 zhǐ (AH$_2$)
趾，在耳尖下方的对耳轮上脚后上部，即对耳轮 2 区。

4.3.3 踝 huái (AH$_3$)
踝，在趾、跟区下方处，即对耳轮 3 区。

4.3.4 膝 xī (AH$_4$)
膝，在对耳轮上脚中 1/3 处，即对耳轮 4 区。

4.3.5 髋 kuān (AH$_5$)
髋，在对耳轮上脚的下 1/3 处，即对耳轮 5 区。

4.3.6 坐骨神经 zuògǔshénjīng (AH$_6$)
坐骨神经，在对耳轮下脚的前 2/3 处，即对耳轮 6 区。

4.3.7 交感 jiāogǎn (AH$_{6a}$)
交感，在对耳轮下脚前端与耳轮内缘交界处，即对耳轮 6 区前端。

4.3.8 臀 tún (AH$_7$)
臀，在对耳轮下脚的后 1/3 处，即对耳轮 7 区。

4.3.9 腹 fù (AH$_8$)
腹，在对耳轮体前部上 2/5 处，即对耳轮 8 区。

4.3.10 腰骶椎 yāodǐzhuī (AH$_9$)
腰骶椎，在腹区后方，即对耳轮 9 区。

4.3.11 胸 xiōng (AH$_{10}$)
胸，在对耳轮体前部中 2/5 处，即对耳轮 10 区。

4.3.12 胸椎 xiōngzhuī (AH$_{11}$)
胸椎，在胸区后方，即对耳轮 11 区。

4.3.13 颈 jǐng (AH$_{12}$)
颈，在对耳轮体前部下 1/5 处，即对耳轮 12 区。

4.3.14 颈椎 jǐngzhuī (AH$_{13}$)
颈椎，在颈区后方，即对耳轮 13 区。

4.4 三角窝穴位

4.4.1 角窝上 jiǎowōshàng (TF$_1$)
角窝上，在三角窝前 1/3 的上部，即三角窝 1 区。

4.4.2 内生殖器 nèishēngzhíqì (TF$_2$)
内生殖器，在三角窝前 1/3 的下部，即三角窝 2 区。

4.4.3 角窝中 jiǎowōzhōng (TF$_3$)
角窝中，在三角窝中 1/3 处，即三角窝 3 区。

4.4.4 神门 shénmén (TF$_4$)
神门，在三角窝后 1/3 的上部，即三角窝 4 区。

4.4.5 盆腔 pénqiāng (TF$_5$)
盆腔，在三角窝后 1/3 的下部，即三角窝 5 区。

4.5 耳屏穴位

4.5.1 上屏 shàngpíng (TG$_1$)

上屏，在耳屏外侧面上 1/2 处，即耳屏 1 区。

4.5.2 下屏 xiàpíng (TG$_2$)

下屏，在耳屏外侧面下 1/2 处，即耳屏 2 区。

4.5.3 外耳 wàiěr (TG$_{1u}$)

外耳，在屏上切迹前方近耳轮部，即耳屏 1 区上缘处。

4.5.4 屏尖 píngjiān (TG$_{1p}$)

屏尖，在耳屏游离缘上部尖端，即耳屏 1 区后缘处。

4.5.5 外鼻 wàibí (TG$_{1,2i}$)

外鼻，在耳屏外侧面中部，即耳屏 1、2 区之间。

4.5.6 肾上腺 shènshàngxiàn (TG$_{2p}$)

肾上腺，在耳屏游离缘下部尖端，即耳屏 2 区后缘处。

4.5.7 咽喉 yānhóu (TG$_3$)

咽喉，在耳屏内侧面上 1/2 处，即耳屏 3 区。

4.5.8 内鼻 nèibí (TG$_4$)

内鼻，在耳屏内侧面下 1/2 处，即耳屏 4 区。

4.5.9 屏间前 píngjiānqián (TG$_{2i}$)

屏间前，在屏间切迹前方耳屏最下部，即耳屏 2 区下缘处。

4.6 对耳屏穴位

4.6.1 额 é (AT$_1$)

额，在对耳屏外侧面的前部，即对耳屏 1 区。

4.6.2 屏间后 píngjiānhòu (AT$_{1i}$)

屏间后，在屏间切迹后方对耳屏前下部，即对耳屏 1 区下缘处。

4.6.3 颞 niè (AT$_2$)

颞，在对耳屏外侧面的中部，即对耳屏 2 区。

4.6.4 枕 zhěn (AT$_3$)

枕，在对耳屏外侧面的后部，即对耳屏 3 区。

4.6.5 皮质下 pízhìxià (AT$_4$)

皮质下，在对耳屏内侧面，即对耳屏 4 区。

4.6.6 对屏尖 duìpíngjiān (AT$_{1,2,4i}$)

对屏尖，在对耳屏游离缘的尖端，即对耳屏 1、2、4 区交点处。

4.6.7 缘中 yuánzhōng (AT$_{2,3,4i}$)

缘中，在对耳屏游离缘上，对屏尖与轮屏切迹之中点处，即对耳屏 2、3、4 区交点处。

4.6.8 脑干 nǎogàn (AT$_{3,4i}$)

脑干，在轮屏切迹处，即对耳屏 3、4 区之间。

4.7 耳甲穴位

4.7.1 口 kǒu (CO$_1$)

口，在耳轮脚下方前 1/3 处，即耳甲 1 区。

4.7.2 食道 shídào (CO$_2$)

食道，在耳轮脚下方中 1/3 处，即耳甲 2 区。

4.7.3　贲门 bēnmén (CO$_3$)

贲门，在耳轮脚下方后 1/3 处，即耳甲 3 区。

4.7.4　胃 wèi (CO$_4$)

胃，在耳轮脚消失处，即耳甲 4 区。

4.7.5　十二指肠 shíèrzhǐcháng (CO$_5$)

十二指肠，在耳轮脚及部分耳轮与 AB 线之间的后 1/3 处，即耳甲 5 区。

4.7.6　小肠 xiǎocháng (CO$_6$)

小肠，在耳轮脚及部分耳轮与 AB 线之间的中 1/3 处，即耳甲 6 区。

4.7.7　大肠 dàcháng (CO$_7$)

大肠，在耳轮脚及部分耳轮与 AB 线之间的前 1/3 处，即耳甲 7 区。

4.7.8　阑尾 lánwěi (CO$_{6,7i}$)

阑尾，在小肠区与大肠区之间，即耳甲 6、7 区交界处。

4.7.9　艇角 tǐngjiǎo (CO$_8$)

艇角，在对耳轮下脚下方前部，即耳甲 8 区。

4.7.10　膀胱 pángguāng (CO$_9$)

膀胱，在对耳轮下脚下方中部，即耳甲 9 区。

4.7.11　肾 shèn (CO$_{10}$)

肾，在对耳轮下脚下方后部，即耳甲 10 区。

4.7.12　输尿管 shūniàoguǎn (CO$_{9,10i}$)

输尿管，在肾区与膀胱区之间，即耳甲 9、10 区交界处。

4.7.13　胰胆 yídǎn (CO$_{11}$)

胰胆，在耳甲艇的后上部，即耳甲 11 区。

4.7.14　肝 gān (CO$_{12}$)

肝，在耳甲艇的后下部，即耳甲 12 区。

4.7.15　艇中 tǐngzhōng (CO$_{6,10i}$)

艇中，在小肠区与肾区之间，即耳甲 6、10 区交界处。

4.7.16　脾 pí (CO$_{13}$)

脾，在 BD 线下方，耳甲腔的后上部，即耳甲 13 区。

4.7.17　心 xīn (CO$_{15}$)

心，在耳甲腔正中凹陷处，即耳甲 15 区。

4.7.18　气管 qìguǎn (CO$_{16}$)

气管，在心区与外耳门之间，即耳甲 16 区。

4.7.19　肺 fèi (CO$_{14}$)

肺，在心、气管区周围处，即耳甲 14 区。

4.7.20　三焦 sānjiāo (CO$_{17}$)

三焦，在外耳门后下，肺与内分泌区之间，即耳甲 17 区。

4.7.21　内分泌 nèifēnmì (CO$_{18}$)

内分泌，在屏间切迹内，耳甲腔的底部，即耳甲 18 区。

4.8　耳垂穴位

4.8.1　牙 yá (LO$_1$)

牙，在耳垂正面前上部，即耳垂 1 区。

4.8.2　舌 shé (LO$_2$)

舌，在耳垂正面中上部，即耳垂 2 区。

4.8.3　颌 hé (LO$_3$)

颌，在耳垂正面后上部，即耳垂 3 区。

4.8.4　垂前 chuíqián (LO$_4$)

垂前，在耳垂正面前中部，即耳垂 4 区。

4.8.5　眼 yǎn (LO$_5$)

眼，在耳垂正面中央部，即耳垂 5 区。

4.8.6　内耳 nèiěr (LO$_6$)

内耳，在耳垂正面后中部，即耳垂 6 区。

4.8.7　面颊 miànjiá (LO$_{5,6i}$)

面颊，在耳垂正面眼区与内耳区之间，即耳垂 5、6 区交界处。

4.8.8　扁桃体 biǎntáotǐ (LO$_{7,8,9}$)

扁桃体，在耳垂正面下部，即耳垂 7、8、9 区。

4.9　耳背穴位

4.9.1　耳背心 ěrbèixīn (P$_1$)

耳背心，在耳背上部，即耳背 1 区。

4.9.2　耳背肺 ěrbèifèi (P$_2$)

耳背肺，在耳背中内部，即耳背 2 区。

4.9.3　耳背脾 ěrbèipí (P$_3$)

耳背脾，在耳背中央部，即耳背 3 区。

4.9.4　耳背肝 ěrbèigān (P$_4$)

耳背肝，在耳背中外部，即耳背 4 区。

4.9.5　耳背肾 ěrbèishèn (P$_5$)

耳背肾，在耳背下部，即耳背 5 区。

4.9.6　耳背沟 ěrbèigōu (P$_s$)

耳背沟，在对耳轮沟和对耳轮上、下脚沟处。

4.10　耳根穴位

4.10.1　上耳根 shàngěrgēn (R$_1$)

上耳根，在耳郭与头部相连的最上处。

4.10.2　耳迷根 ěrmígēn (R$_2$)

耳迷根，在耳轮脚后沟的耳根处。

4.10.3　下耳根 xiàěrgēn (R$_3$)

下耳根，在耳郭与头部相连的最下处。

附录 A

（资料性附录）

耳穴图

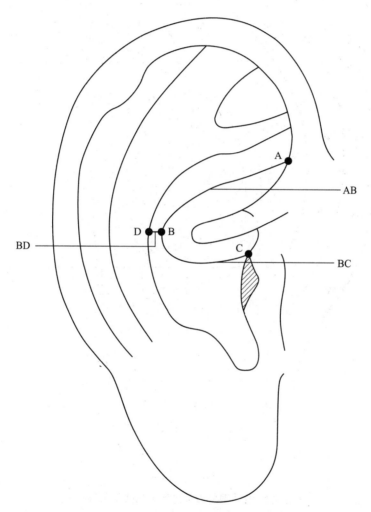

图 A1　补充设定的耳郭标志点或线条示意图

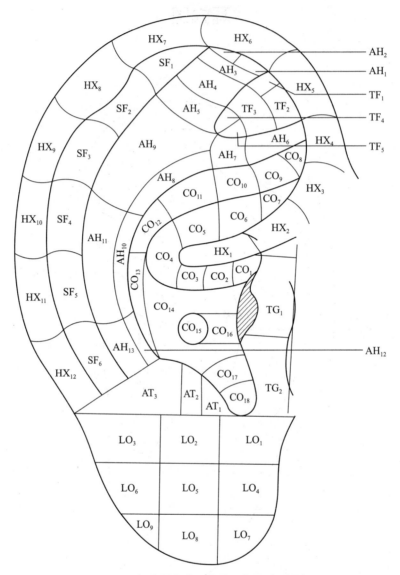

图 A2　标准耳郭分区代号示意图（正面）

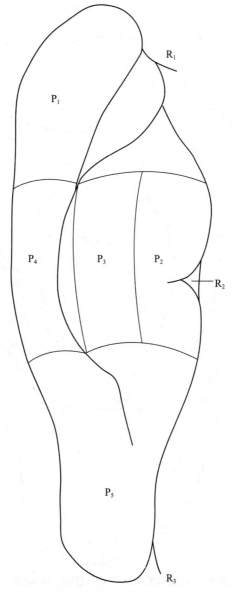

图 A3　标准耳郭分区代号示意图（背面）

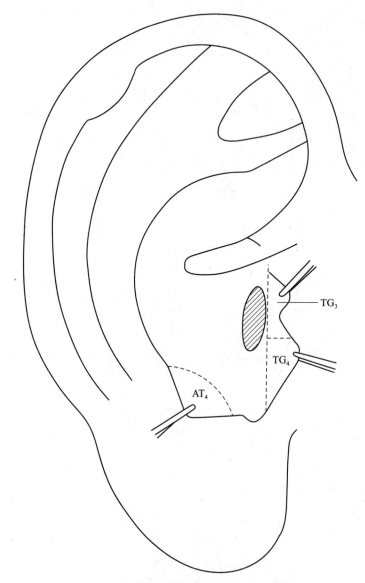

图 A4　标准耳郭分区代号示意图（内侧面）

附录 B

（资料性附录）

耳穴名称与定位命名原则及定位原则

B.1　本标准选取耳穴的原则

B.1.1　有广泛实践基础。

B.1.2　临床上常用的耳穴。

B.1.3　诊疗效果较好的耳穴。

B.2　本标准耳穴命名的原则

　　本标准耳穴命名的原则：在符合上述原则的基础上，还应具备下列特征之一。

B.2.1　目前国际上公认或使用的，如肾上腺、交感等。

B.2.2　见于传统医学文献并经实践证明确有应用价值的，如耳中、耳尖等。

B.2.3　根据人体部位和器官命名的，如心、肩等。

B.2.4　用耳郭解剖术语命名的，如上耳根、角窝中等。

B.2.5　本标准不采用下列方法命名的耳穴。

　　　　a. 以病症术语命名的耳穴名称。

　　　　b. 以某些诊治功能命名的耳穴名称。

　　　　c. 以药物名称命名的耳穴名称。

　　　　d. 与入选本标准耳穴处于同一穴位区域内的其他耳穴名称。

　　　　e. 具有性别特征的耳穴名称。

　　　　f. 其他不符合入选特征的耳穴名称。

B.3　耳穴名称与定位原则

B.3.1　本标准采用以分区定位为主，区、点结合的方法定位。

B.3.2　明确规定表示耳郭位置的名词术语。

B.3.3　介绍与耳穴分区定位有关的耳郭表面解剖名称。

B.3.4　根据耳郭表面解剖结构补充设立若干耳穴定位标志点。

B.3.5　划定耳郭基本标志线，标清各解剖结构之分野，在各部位结构的基础上以解剖标志分区标定穴位。

B.3.6　穴位（区）覆盖全部耳郭表面。

附录 C

（资料性附录）

耳郭基本标志点、线的划定及耳郭分区说明

C.1 耳郭基本标志线的划定

下列耳郭基本标志线的划定适用于耳郭分区的说明。

C.1.1 耳轮内缘

耳轮内缘，即耳轮与耳郭其他部分的分界线，指耳轮与耳舟、对耳轮上脚、对耳轮下脚、三角窝及耳甲等部的折线。

C.1.2 耳甲折线

耳甲折线，指耳甲内平坦部与隆起部之间的折线。

C.1.3 对耳轮脊线

对耳轮脊线，指对耳轮体及其上、下脚最凸起处之连线。

C.1.4 耳舟凹沟线

耳舟凹沟线，指沿耳舟最凹陷处所做的连线。

C.1.5 对耳轮耳舟缘

对耳轮耳舟缘，即对耳轮与耳舟的分界线，指对耳轮（含对耳轮上脚）脊与耳舟凹沟之间的中线。

C.1.6 三角窝凹陷处后缘

三角窝凹陷处后缘，指三角窝内较低平的三角形区域的后缘。

C.1.7 对耳轮三角窝缘

对耳轮三角窝缘，即对耳轮上、下脚与三角窝的分界线，指对耳轮上、下脚脊与三角窝凹陷处后缘之间的中线。

C.1.8 对耳轮耳甲缘

对耳轮耳甲缘，即对耳轮与耳甲的分界线，指对耳轮（含对耳轮下脚）脊与耳甲折线之间的中线。

C.1.9 对耳轮上脚下缘

对耳轮上脚下缘，即对耳轮上脚与对耳轮体的分界线，指从对耳轮上、下脚分叉处向对耳轮耳舟缘所做的垂线。

C.1.10 对耳轮下脚后缘

对耳轮下脚后缘，即对耳轮下脚与对耳轮体的分界线，指从对耳轮上、下脚分叉处向对耳轮耳甲缘所做的垂线。

C.1.11 耳垂上线

耳垂上线，即耳垂与耳郭其他部分的分界线，指过屏间切迹与轮垂切迹所做的直线。

C.1.12 对耳屏耳甲缘

对耳屏耳甲缘，即对耳轮与耳甲的分界线，指对耳屏内侧面与耳甲的折线。

C.1.13 耳屏前缘

耳屏前缘，即耳屏外侧面与面部的分界线，指沿耳屏前沟所做的直线。

C.1.14 耳轮前缘

耳轮前缘，即耳轮与面部的分界线，指沿耳轮前沟所做的直线。

C.1.15 耳垂前缘

耳垂前缘，即耳垂与面颊的分界线，指沿耳垂前沟所做的直线。

C.2 耳郭标志点、线的设定

下列耳郭基本标志点、线的划定适用于耳郭分区的说明。

C.2.1 在耳轮内缘上，设耳轮脚切迹至对耳轮下脚间中、上 1/3 交界处为 A 点。

C.2.2 在耳甲内，由耳轮脚消失处向后做一水平线与对耳轮耳甲缘相交，设交点为 D 点。

C.2.3 设耳轮脚消失处至 D 点连线的中、后 1/3 交界处为 B 点。

C.2.4 设外耳道口后缘上 1/4 与下 3/4 交界处为 C 点。

C.2.5 从 A 点向 B 点做一条与对耳轮耳甲艇缘弧度大体相仿的曲线。

C.2.6 从 B 点向 C 点做一条与耳轮脚下缘弧度大体相仿的曲线。

C.3 耳郭分区的说明

C.3.1 耳轮

耳轮脚为耳轮 1 区；耳轮脚切迹到对耳轮下脚上缘之间的耳轮分为三等分，自下而上依次为耳轮 2 区、耳轮 3 区、耳轮 4 区；对耳轮下脚上缘到对耳轮上脚前缘之间的耳轮为耳轮 5 区；对耳轮上脚前缘到耳尖之间的耳轮为耳轮 6 区；耳尖到耳轮结节上缘为耳轮 7 区；耳轮结节上缘到耳轮结节下缘为耳轮 8 区；耳轮结节下缘到轮垂切迹之间的耳轮分为 4 等分，自上而下依次为耳轮 9 区、耳轮 10 区、耳轮 11 区、耳轮 12 区。

C.3.2 耳舟

耳舟分为 6 等分，自上而下依次为耳舟 1 区、耳舟 2 区、耳舟 3 区、耳舟 4 区、耳舟 5 区、耳舟 6 区。

C.3.3 对耳轮

对耳轮上脚分为上、中、下 3 等分，下 1/3 为对耳轮 5 区，中 1/3 为对耳轮 4 区；再将上 1/3 分为上、下 2 等分，下 1/2 为对耳轮 3 区；再将上 1/2 分为前、后 2 等分，后 1/2 为对耳轮 2 区，前 1/2 为对耳轮 1 区。

对耳轮下脚分为前、中、后 3 等分，中、前 2/3 为对耳轮 6 区，后 1/3 为对耳轮 7 区。

将对耳轮体从对耳轮上、下脚分叉处至轮屏切迹分为 5 等分，再沿对耳轮耳甲缘将对耳轮体分为前 1/4 和后 3/4 两部分，前上 2/5 为对耳轮 8 区，后上 2/5 为对耳轮 9 区，前中 2/5 为对耳轮 10 区，后中 2/5 为对耳轮 11 区，前下 1/5 为对耳轮 12 区，后下 1/5 为对耳轮 13 区。

C.3.4 三角窝

将三角窝由耳轮内缘至对耳轮上、下脚分叉处分为前、中、后 3 等分，中 1/3 为三角窝 3 区；再将前 1/3 分为上、中、下 3 等分，上 1/3 为三角窝 1 区，中、下 2/3 为三角窝 2 区；再将后 1/3 分为上、下 2 等分，上 1/2 为三角窝 4 区，下 1/2 为三角窝 5 区。

C.3.5 耳屏

将耳屏外侧面分为上、下 2 等分，上部为耳屏 1 区，下部为耳屏 2 区。

将耳屏内侧面分为上、下 2 等分，上部为耳屏 3 区，下部为耳屏 4 区。

C.3.6 对耳屏

由对屏尖及对屏尖至轮屏切迹连线之中点，分别向耳垂上线做两条垂线，将对耳屏外侧面及其后部分为前、中、后三区，前为对耳屏 1 区，中为对耳屏 2 区，后为对耳屏 3 区。

对耳屏内侧面为对耳屏 4 区。

C.3.7 耳甲

将 BC 线前段与耳轮脚下缘间分成 3 等分，前 1/3 为耳甲 1 区，中 1/3 为耳甲 2 区，后 1/3 为耳甲 3 区。

ABC 线前方，耳轮脚消失处为耳甲 4 区。

将 AB 线前段与耳轮脚上缘及部分耳轮内缘间分成 3 等分，后 1/3 为耳甲 5 区，中 1/3 为耳甲 6 区，前 1/3 为耳甲 7 区。

将对耳轮下脚下缘前、中 1/3 交界处与 C 点连线，该线前方的耳甲艇部为耳甲 8 区。

将 AB 线前段与对耳轮下脚下缘间耳甲 8 区以后的部分，分为前、后 2 等分，前 1/2 为耳甲 9 区，后 1/2 为耳甲 10 区。

在 AB 线后段上方的耳甲艇部，将耳甲 10 区后缘与 BD 线之间分成上、下 2 等分，上 1/2 为耳甲 11 区，下 1/2 为耳甲 12 区。

由轮屏切迹至 B 点做连线，该线后方、BD 线下方的耳甲腔部为耳甲 13 区。

以耳甲腔中央为圆心，圆心与 BC 线间距离的 1/2 为半径做圆，该圆形区域为耳甲 15 区。

过耳甲 15 区的最高点及最低点分别向外耳门后壁做两条切线，切线间为耳甲 16 区。

耳甲 15 区、耳甲 16 区周围为耳甲 14 区。

将外耳门的最低点与对耳屏耳甲缘中点相连，再将该线以下的耳甲腔部分为上、下 2 等分，上 1/2 为耳甲 17 区，下 1/2 为耳甲 18 区。

C.3.8 耳垂

在耳垂上线至耳垂下缘最低点之间画两条等距离的平行线，于上平行线上引两条垂直等分线，将耳垂分为 9 个区。上部由前到后依次为耳垂 1 区、耳垂 2 区、耳垂 3 区；中部由前到后依次为耳垂 4 区、耳垂 5 区、耳垂 6 区；下部由前到后依次为耳垂 7 区、耳垂 8 区、耳垂 9 区。

C.3.9 耳背

分别过对耳轮上、下脚分叉处耳背对应点和轮屏切迹耳背对应点做两条水平线，将耳背分为上、中、下三部，上部为耳背 1 区，下部为耳背 5 区；再将中部分为内、中、外 3 等分，内 1/3 为耳背 2 区，中 1/3 为耳背 3 区，外 1/3 为耳背 4 区。

———————